"Remember

To: Lily
with love!

Remember Me...
Remember Me Not

Carma Lee Weisbrook *Carma Lee*
Illustrated by Susan Shorter *Weisbrook*

AuthorHouse™ LLC
1663 Liberty Drive
Bloomington, IN 47403
www.authorhouse.com
Phone: 1-800-839-8640

© 2014 Carma Lee Weisbrook. All rights reserved.

No part of this book may be reproduced, stored in a retrieval system, or transmitted by any means without the written permission of the author.

Published by AuthorHouse 05/30/2014

ISBN: 978-1-4969-1469-9 (sc)
ISBN: 978-1-4969-1468-2 (e)

Library of Congress Control Number: 2014909339

Any people depicted in stock imagery provided by Thinkstock are models, and such images are being used for illustrative purposes only.
Certain stock imagery © Thinkstock.

This book is printed on acid-free paper.

Because of the dynamic nature of the Internet, any web addresses or links contained in this book may have changed since publication and may no longer be valid. The views expressed in this work are solely those of the author and do not necessarily reflect the views of the publisher, and the publisher hereby disclaims any responsibility for them.

Me, mom, and my sister

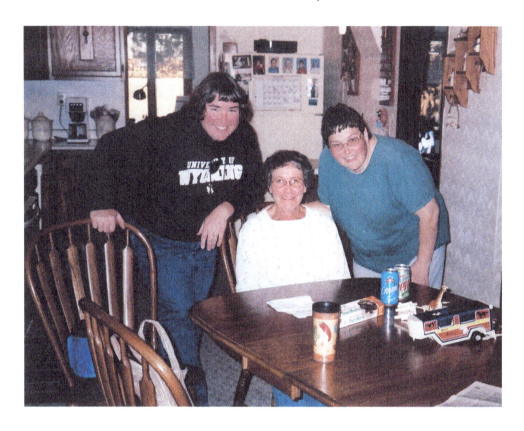

This book is dedicated to my mom.

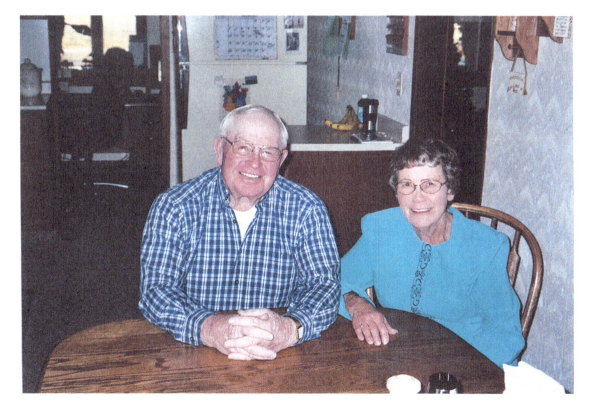

My parents, married 54 years

As the early morning sunlight streamed into the bedroom, I jumped out of bed and shouted, "Today is the big day!" All of the red X's on the calendar confirmed the fact that this day marked the beginning of my week with Grandma. After pulling on jean shorts and a bright-yellow T-shirt, I raced to the kitchen. My mother and I quickly ate fresh fruit and yogurt for breakfast, loaded my suitcase into the car, and hit the familiar road to Grandma's house.

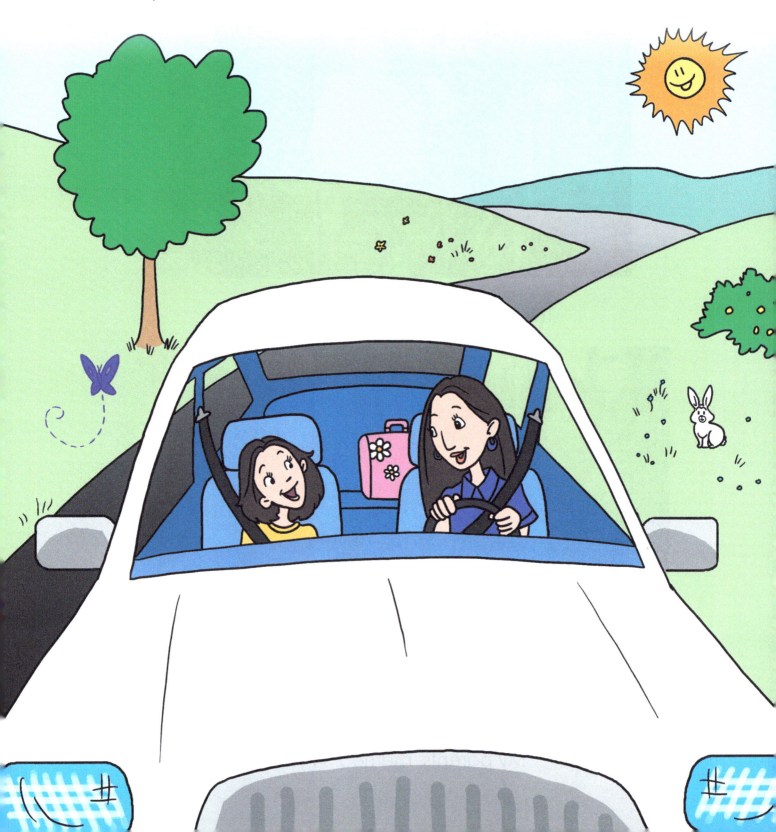

"How many more miles, Mom? I cannot wait to get to Grandma's house!"

"I know, Jodi, you have been waiting and waiting for fourth grade to be finished so you can go visit Grandma," stated Mom as we rounded the corner. "What is your favorite thing to do at Grandma's house?"

"I love to feed the birds and work in the flower garden. I hope we can play this game that Grandma taught me last summer."

"What game is that?" Mom inquired.

"We picked one of Grandma's flowers—a daisy, I think. We pulled off one petal at a time and said, 'She loves me. She loves me not.' And we just laughed and laughed."

"We are here," Mom announced as she put the car into park. I ran for the house.

We found Grandma inside the house, resting. She looked older than I remembered. Mom had to wake her. Did she forget we were coming today?

"Hello, Julie," was her sleepy reply.

"Grandma, I am Jodi. You called me by my mom's name," I whispered.

"Of course, I remember now. It is good to see you both. Let's go have some tea," Grandma said.

While the adults chatted, I was anxious for my mom to leave so that we could begin our busy week.

"Do you have everything, Jodi?" Mom asked as she prepared to leave.

"Yes, Mom, I do."

"It is going to be a quiet week without you." After a hug and a kiss, Mom was off. "Have a great week you two!" Mom shouted as she disappeared around the bend.

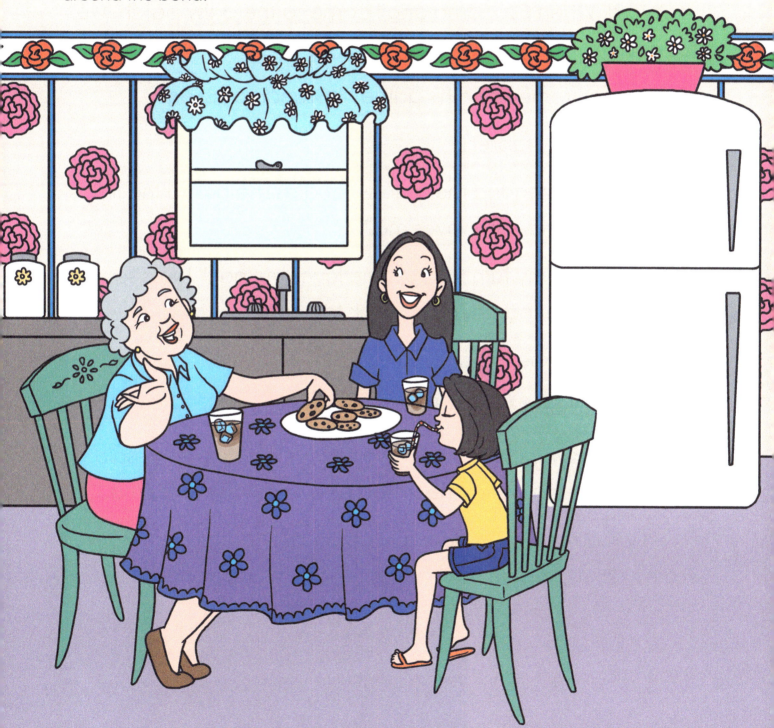

"I have looked forward to this for a long time!"

"Me too," Grandma replied.

We walked hand in hand to the flower garden in the backyard. When Grandma and I came to the daisy patch, we stopped.

"Do you remember this game?" Grandma asked.

"I sure do!" I replied.

Grandma handed me a daisy, and as she pulled the first petal off, she said, "She loves me."

It was now my turn to say, "She loves me not." I was so happy; our time together was back to normal.

"She loves me," Grandma sang.

I giggled and said, "She loves me not."

"You know that Grandma will always love you," she said. Pulling off the last petal, she smiled and said, "She loves me."

"I will always love you too, Grandma." After our game, we walked slowly, beside each other to sit in the cool shade.

"Goodness, I get so tired these days," Grandma stated as she sat down in her lawn chair. In no time at all, Jodi noticed that Grandma was asleep.

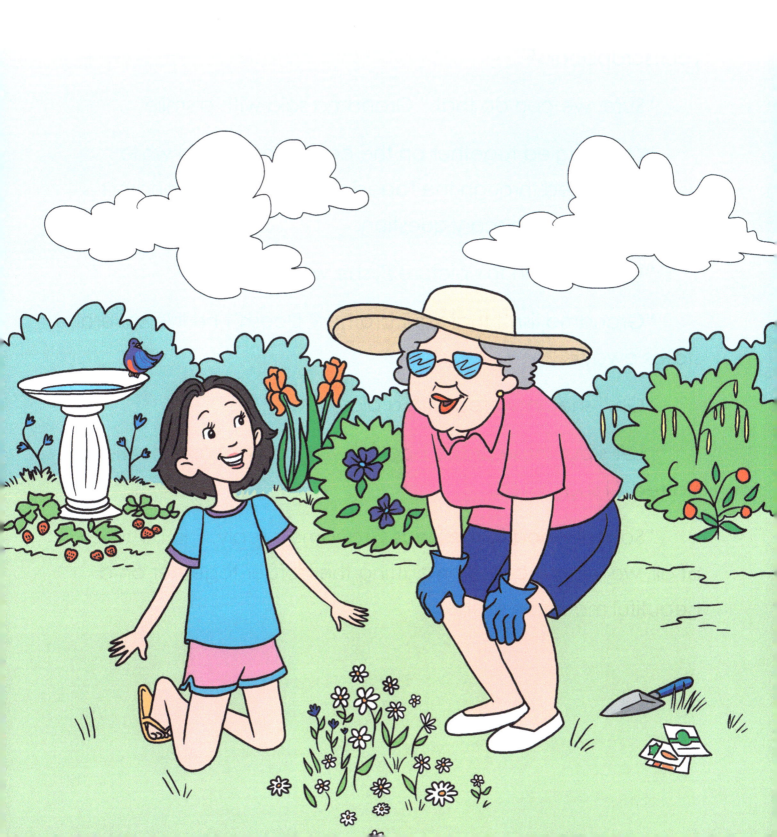

After her nap, I asked, "Grandma, can we look through your scrapbooks?"

"Sure, we can do that," Grandma said with a smile.

We snuggled together on the couch for quite a while as we thumbed through the faded pictures. Then Grandma shocked me with a scary question.

"Who is that in this picture?" she wondered.

"Grandma, isn't that your brother? Doesn't he live several states away?"

"Oh," she answered with a blank stare.

"Let's put these photo books away and get us a puzzle started," I suggested.

"Sounds good to me" was Grandma's reply. In no time at all, we were focused on putting the border together on a beautiful mountain scene.

Gorgeous summer weather greeted us the next day.

"It's a great day to work in the garden!" Grandma announced as we finished the breakfast dishes. "I'll be right back. I am going to get our garden gloves from the garage." After several minutes went by, I began to get worried about Grandma, so I went to look for her. I found her seated in the garage and very upset.

"Grandma, what is wrong? Are you hurt?" I asked while I grabbed Grandma and hugged her.

"Oh, there you are. Why did I come into the garage?" Grandma wondered.

"You came to get our garden gloves so that we can go to the flower garden," I replied as I tried not to panic.

"Oh, that is right. I forgot," Grandma confessed. "It must be my old age because I keep forgetting a lot lately."

"Can we go to the garden now?" I asked.

"Sure" was Grandma's quiet response.

Grandma seemed so confused. I reminded myself to tell Mom about this later.

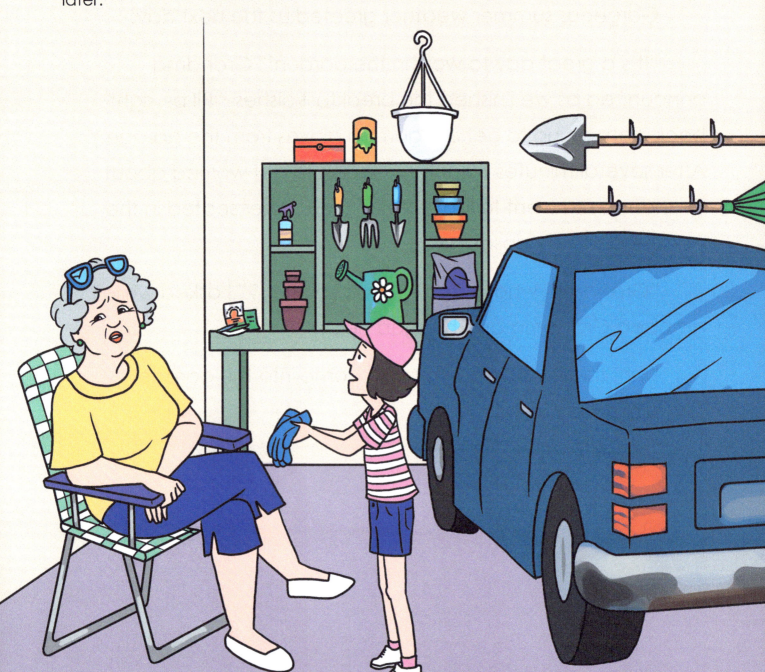

The week went by quickly. Grandma and I had a great time. Soon, Mom came to spend a few days with us.

"Mom's here," I shouted as I ran for the driveway.

"Hello, Kathy," Grandma said as she greeted her daughter.

"Mom, I am Julie, not Kathy. She lives in Colorado," said my mom with a rather confused look on her face. "How was your week with Jodi?"

"It was wonderful!" Grandma replied with a big smile.

"Mom, Grandma, come have some tea. I made it myself," I proudly stated as the two of them came inside.

"Mom, I think it is time for you to have a checkup. I made an appointment with your family doctor. He can see you this afternoon," my mother stated.

"I suppose," Grandma replied. After a fresh salad of greens and strawberries from the garden, we left to see the family doctor.

When Grandma's name was called, Mom said, "Please wait here. Find a magazine to read. We will be right back."

"All right, Mom," I said, already skimming the stack of magazines.

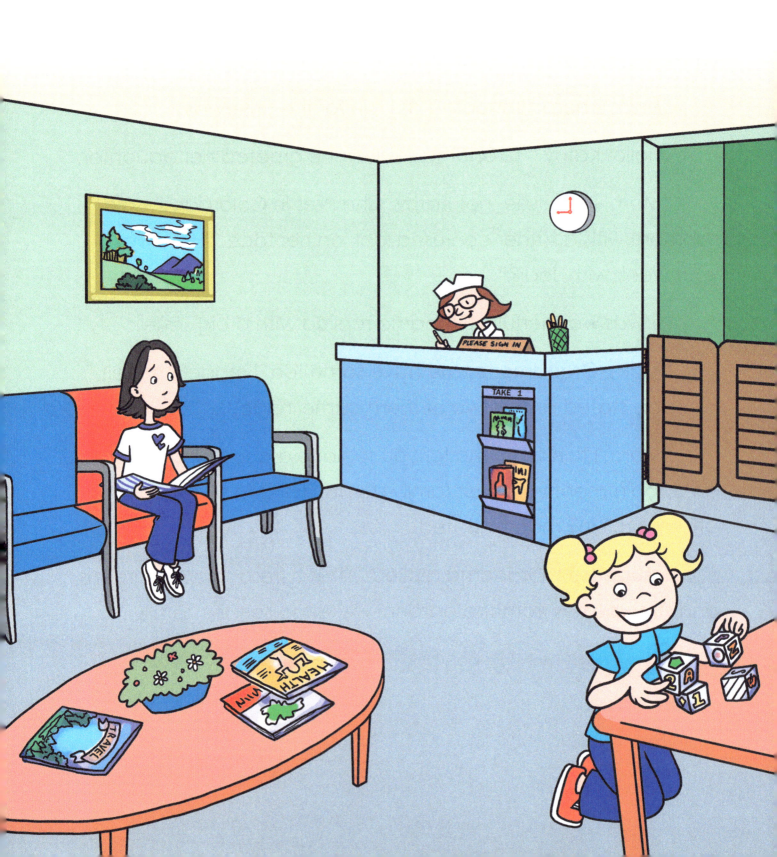

Mom and Grandma were in with the doctor for a long time. When they came out, they both appeared very sad.

"Mom! What is wrong?" I inquired.

"Let's get in the car. We will talk about it later." The ride from the doctor's office was a long one. All of us rode in silence. I was getting more concerned with every passing moment. Did the news from the doctor have something to do with Grandma calling family members by the wrong names? What about her forgetting things? I held these thoughts inside my head as we drove quietly to Grandma's home.

When we got to her house, Grandma broke the silence with this question: "What is Alzheimer's disease?"

"Alzheimer's?" I said in a demanding tone. "Is that what the doctor told Grandma she might have? What is that?"

"Well, Jodi, it is a disease of the brain," Mom explained.

"*No!*" I screamed. I ran to the garden, crying. I did not want my grandma to have a disease. Why did this have to happen?

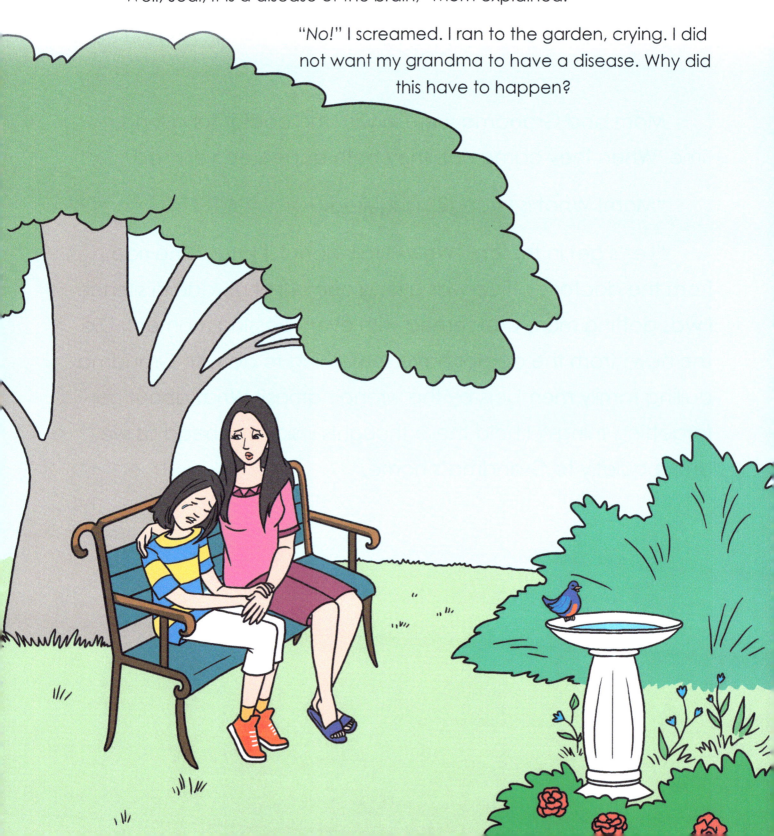

A short time later, Mom quietly joined me in the garden. She sat down beside me and placed her arm around me. We sat there for a long time.

"Grandma is resting after her long afternoon, so I wanted to come and talk to you. Do you know anything about Alzheimer's disease?" she asked me.

"No. I have heard of it, but I do not know what it is," I replied.

"It is a disease of the brain. That is why Grandma is having such a hard time remembering these days," Mom explained.

"She forgot why she went into the garage. She also forgot who her brother was in a picture," I explained.

"Yes, I am so glad that you told me. The doctor says that there is some medicine he can give her," Mom explained.

"Good. So Grandma will get better?" I asked.

"No, I am sorry, Jodi. There is no cure for this disease. Sadly, Grandma will continue to get steadily worse," Mom said, tears in her eyes.

"Worse? What do you mean?" I asked.

"The doctor says that she cannot live alone anymore. She must be in a place where there are nurses at all times," explained Mom.

"Why? Why did Grandma have to get this?" I screamed.

"There is no explanation for disease. This is an awful thing that we must live with. We must be strong for Grandma and help her. Can you promise me that you will help?" Mom asked.

"I will help," I replied.

The next few months included many changes. Grandma had to move away from her home in the country to a facility. It was very difficult for all of us. Grandma adjusted slowly to her new place, and she enjoyed it when I came to see her.

"I brought you a daisy, Grandma," I announced after entering her room.

"She loves me," I started.

"She loves me not," Grandma said.

"She loves me," I repeated.

"She loves me not," Grandma said. "But that is not true. I will always love you, Jodi!"

"I know, Grandma. I will always love you too."

I snuggled in close to Grandma and silently sat on the couch.

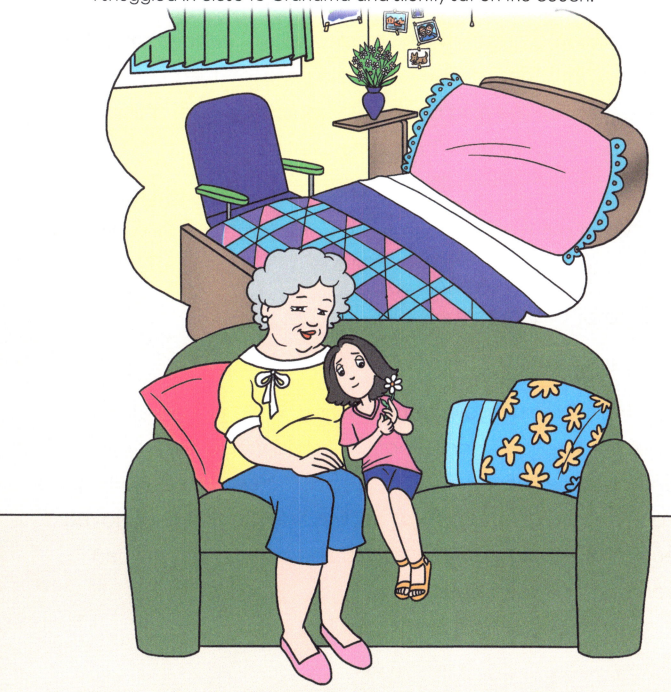

One day, I was on my way to see Grandma. It was a nice day, and I planned to have the nurse help me take her outside.

"Are you Jodi?" the nurse asked with a big smile.

"Yes, I am," I whispered. "Who are you?"

"I am your grandma's nurse. She talks about you all the time," she said. "What is the game that you play with her? The game with the flowers?"

"Grandma and I play this game called 'she loves me, she loves me not.' The first time you pull a petal off the daisy, say, 'She loves me.' The next person who pulls a petal off the daisy says, 'She loves me not.' The game continues until all the petals are gone."

"What a fun game," the nurse commented as we went our different ways.

"Hello, Grandma."

"Hello, Kathy," Grandma misspoke.

"Hello," I said again, remembering not to get upset. Having Alzheimer's disease meant that Grandma would forget my name, but she knew I was very special to her. After a short visit, I could tell that Grandma was getting tired, so I told her I loved her and quietly tiptoed out. I was sitting on the bench when Grandma's nurse spotted me.

"Jodi?" she quietly said.

"Yes," I said, wiping the tears from my eyes.

"Are you all right?" she asked.

"No, I am not! I am so sad. It is just not fair!" I screamed.

"I understand, Jodi," the nurse whispered. "I have worked here for many years, and it is an awful disease.

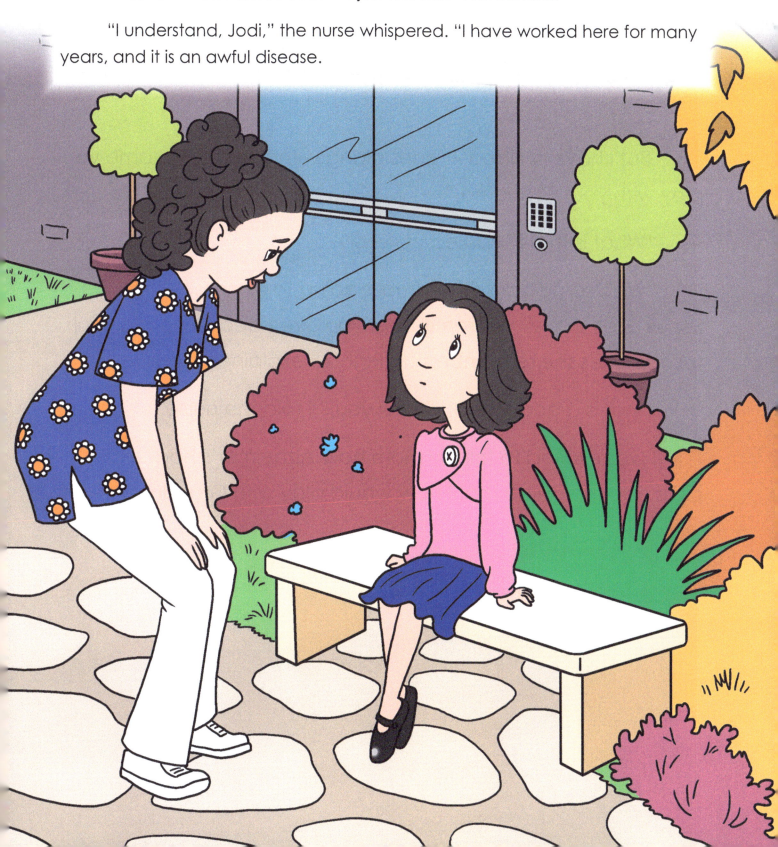

But I have an idea. It goes along with the flower game you play with your Grandma."

"What is that?" I asked curiously.

"Well, some days Grandma is going to remember you. Some days she will not remember you. We need to be thankful for the times she remembers us. Right?" explained the nurse.

"That is a good idea. Thank you," I told the nurse.

I was excited to tell my mom how Alzheimer's had changed the game that I now would play with Grandma.

"How was Grandma?" she asked.

"She seemed so tired today," I said.

"We will go see her again very soon," Mom replied.

"I have a new way to play our game, Mom," I said "Grandma's nurse taught it to me. It goes like this: she remembers me, she remembers me not. The nurse taught me that we are to be thankful for the times she remembers us."

"Wonderful," Mom said, proudly smiling.

"But one thing is for certain. We will *always* love Grandma, no matter what!"

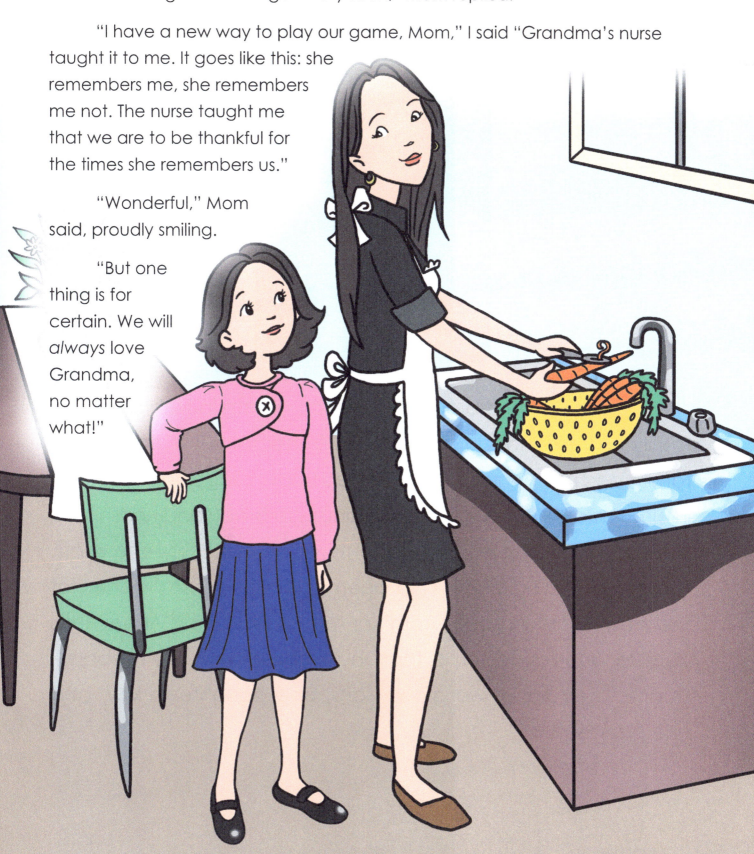

About the Author

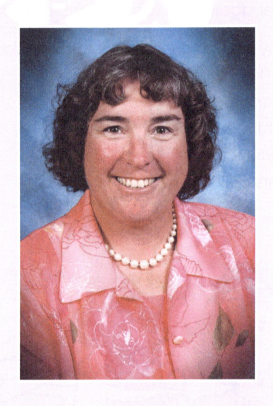

Carma Lee Weisbrook grew up on a farm in Nebraska. Her family and extended family instilled in her faith in God, love of family, and hard work. She graduated from college with a degree in elementary education. She continues to teach and has shared her love of learning with her students for the past thirty-one years. She enjoys writing stories and poems about her family. She got the idea for her first book from her mother, who had Alzheimer's disease. She resides on a farm in Nebraska with her husband, Duane. They have two grown sons, one daughter-in-law, and one grandson.

CPSIA information can be obtained at www.ICGtesting.com
Printed in the USA
LVOW02s0457250614

391607LV00003B/16/P